7 Keys to Divine Health

Emmanuel AnuOluwatomiwa

Table of Content

Introduction

Divine health doesn't mean living without health challenges; it means overcoming them through the power of what's already been done for us—1 Peter 2:24. Our bodies aren't fully redeemed yet, so they can still be vulnerable to attacks. However, we can decide what our bodies respond to— whether it's the Word of God or disease-causing agents.

Just as children can be trained to communicate when they need to use the restroom, we can train our bodies to respond only to what is aligned with God's Word. This explains why people living in the same environment can have different health experiences.

Living in divine health is about establishing a mindset and lifestyle that aligns with God's promises. It is not a passive state but an active engagement with spiritual truths and practices. Divine health means standing firm on the belief that God's will for us is to be healthy and whole, regardless of the physical symptoms that may try to challenge this truth. It is about adopting a holistic approach that includes both spiritual and practical steps to maintain a state of wellness.

The journey to divine health begins with renewing our minds (Romans 12:2). This transformation involves feeding on God's Word until it becomes more real to us than any diagnosis or symptom. It's about letting go of fear, doubt, and unbelief and embracing faith, hope, and love. When our thoughts and beliefs are aligned with God's promises, our bodies will eventually follow suit.

Furthermore, it is crucial to understand that divine health is not just about physical well-being. It encompasses mental, emotional, and spiritual health. God's desire is for us to prosper and be in good health, even as our soul prospers (3 John 1:2). This means that a balanced life, filled with peace, joy, and a sound mind, is integral to experiencing divine health.

In this book, we will explore the seven keys to achieving and maintaining divine health. Each key represents a principle or practice that, when consistently applied, can unlock the door to a life of vibrant health and vitality. From speaking life-giving words to making wise dietary choices, from walking in love and forgiveness to guarding your heart against negative influences—each key plays a vital role in creating an environment where divine health can flourish.

As you read through these pages, I encourage you to keep an open heart and a willing spirit. Let the truths shared here inspire you to take bold steps of faith toward divine health. Remember, this is not just about reading another book; it's about experiencing a transformation in your health journey. The power to live in divine health is already within you, waiting to be activated by faith and obedience to God's Word.

Let's embark on this journey together and discover the keys to divine health that God has graciously provided for us. Your best health is yet to come!

"He himself bore our sins in his body on the tree, that we might die to sin and live to righteousness. By his wounds you have been healed." 1 Pet. 2:24

The same sacrifice for your sin settled your healing.

Chapter 1

You Were Not Created to Be Sick

Man was not originally created to experience sickness or death. In the beginning, God designed a perfect world where Adam and Eve lived in harmony with God, each other, and all creation. Sickness was never part of God's original plan. Healing only became necessary after the fall, when sin entered the world, bringing with it spiritual, mental, and physical death.

Spiritual Death

When Adam sinned, he experienced spiritual death first, which is directly tied to the withdrawal of God's light. John 1:3-4 tells us, ***"Through Him, all things were made; without Him, nothing was made that has been made. In Him was life, and that life was the light of all mankind."*** This light represents the divine presence of God, His life, and His sustaining power. The moment Adam sinned, the life of God—manifested as light—departed from him. Darkness, which symbolizes separation from God, immediately overshadowed him, and the pangs of this darkness began to take their toll. This spiritual death was not just a separation from God's presence, but also from His life-giving light, leaving Adam vulnerable to the powers of darkness and the agents of death, such as sickness.

Before the fall, Adam walked in the light of God's presence, but after sin entered, he was plunged into darkness. Genesis 3:8-9 captures this tragic shift when Adam and Eve hid from God among the trees of the garden. God's question, **"Where are you?"** was not just about their physical location, but also about their spiritual condition. Their inner light had been extinguished, leading to fear, shame, and a loss of their original spiritual vitality.

Darkness became the new reality for humanity, and this darkness gave rise to all kinds of evil, including sickness and disease. Without the protective light of God, Adam's body was left exposed to the buffeting of agents of death—sickness being one of the primary manifestations. However, through Christ, the light has returned to us. John 8:12 says, ***"I am the light of the world. Whoever follows me will never walk in darkness, but will have the light of life."*** Through Jesus, we have been restored to God's light, which brings healing and wholeness to every part of our being.

Mental Death

Adam's fall also affected his mental faculties. Originally, Adam was so mentally sharp and wise that God entrusted him with the task of naming every living creature (Genesis 2:19-20). Imagine the level of intellect and creativity required to name every animal, bird, and fish! Adam's mind was in perfect harmony with God's, enabling him to perform this immense task with divine insight. But after the fall, Adam's mental clarity was clouded. The first thing he did after realizing he was naked was to sew fig leaves together to cover himself and Eve (Genesis 3:7). This was an inadequate and temporary solution, revealing a diminished capacity to solve problems.

This deterioration in mental sharpness illustrates what we could call "mental death." When we are disconnected from God, our thinking becomes futile, and our understanding darkened (Ephesians 4:18). We start making decisions based on fear, insecurity, and pride, rather than divine wisdom. But the good news is that through Christ, our minds can be renewed. Romans 12:2 says, **"*Do not conform to the pattern of this world, but be transformed by the renewing of your mind.*"** When we allow God's Word to renew our minds, we can think clearly and make decisions aligned with His will.

Physical Death

Finally, Adam's body, which was initially designed for eternal life, became susceptible to sickness and death. While God's gifts and call are irrevocable (Romans 11:29), the entrance of sin meant that physical death became an inevitability. God had warned Adam that eating from the tree of the knowledge of good and evil would result in death (Genesis 2:17). And so it was—Adam's body began to age and eventually succumbed to death. Sickness is a manifestation of this process. It is the body's gradual decline and eventual death sentence.

Romans 6:23 reminds us, **"*For the wages of sin is death, but the gift of God is eternal life in Christ Jesus our Lord.*"** Sin's goal is ultimately to bring about death, but Jesus came to give us life—abundant life (John 10:10). This includes physical health and wholeness. Jesus' ministry on earth was marked by healing the sick, raising the dead, and casting out demons, demonstrating God's will for His people to live in divine health. In Matthew 8:17, we read that Jesus healed the sick to fulfill what was spoken by the prophet Isaiah: **"*He took up our infirmities and bore our diseases.*"**

The Path to Restoration

Though man fell from his original state of divine health, God has provided a way back through Jesus Christ. Our salvation includes not just spiritual renewal but also healing for our minds and bodies. Isaiah 53:5 declares, **"*But He was pierced for our transgressions, He was crushed for our iniquities; the punishment that brought us peace was on Him, and by His wounds, we are healed.*"** This means that divine health is available to us today. Through Christ, we can reclaim the health and wholeness that was originally ours.

To live in divine health, we must first recognize that we were not created to be sick. Sickness is an intruder, a byproduct of the fall. We must also understand that Jesus has already made provision for our healing. It's time to renew our minds, align our thoughts with God's Word, and exercise our faith to walk in the divine health that has been made available to us through Christ.

The choice is ours: Will we accept sickness as a natural part of life, or will we stand on the promises of God, believing in His best? Remember, you were not created to be sick. Your inheritance as a child of God is divine health, and through Christ, you have the authority to claim it.

"He himself bore our sins in his body on the tree, that we might die to sin and live to righteousness. By his wounds you have been healed." 1 Pet. 2:24

The same sacrifice for your sin settled your healing.

Chapter 2

Medicine is Not Evil

In our journey toward divine health, it is essential to understand that medical treatments and drugs are not evil; they are, in fact, a part of God's provision to sustain life while we build our faith in divine healing. As John 3:27 reminds us, **_A man can receive nothing unless it has been given to him from heaven._** Medical knowledge and interventions are gifts from God, tools He has provided to help us navigate life's challenges, including health issues.

Medicine as a Gift from God

It's important to dispel the myth that using medicine means you lack faith or have sinned against God. Throughout the Bible, we see examples of God using various means to bring healing, including natural remedies and even physicians. Consider Hezekiah, the king of Judah, who was healed after applying a poultice of figs as instructed by the prophet Isaiah (Isaiah 38:21). This story illustrates that God can use both natural remedies and supernatural means to heal. If God were against medical interventions, He would not have instructed the king to apply the poultice.

God's provision of medicine and medical professionals is another expression of His love and grace towards humanity. The Bible speaks positively about physicians. Jesus Himself acknowledged the role of doctors when He said, **_It is not_** *the healthy who need a doctor, but the sick"* (Luke 5:31). This statement underscores that while divine healing is available, medical intervention is a valid and necessary part of caring for the body.

A Balanced Perspective on Faith and Medicine

Faith in God's healing power and the use of medicine are not mutually exclusive. You can believe in divine healing while also using medicine to manage symptoms or aid recovery. God works in many ways, and His ways are higher than ours (Isaiah 55:9). Sometimes, He may choose to heal instantaneously; other times, He may use medicine or a medical professional.

It is vital to understand that taking medicine does not imply a lack of faith. James 2:17 teaches us that *"faith by itself, if it is not accompanied by action, is dead."* In many instances, taking medicine is the action step we take while standing in faith for complete healing. It demonstrates our willingness to do our part while trusting God to do His. After all, medicine can treat symptoms, but ultimate healing comes from God alone.

Knowledge and Wisdom in Health Decisions

It's also important to base your health beliefs and actions on sound knowledge and personal revelation, not on hearsay or misconceptions. Proverbs 4:7 tells us, *"Wisdom is the principal thing; therefore get wisdom: and with all thy getting, get understanding."* God has given us wisdom, and part of that wisdom is understanding how to use the resources available to us, including medicine, to maintain our health.

One of the mistakes many believers make is to lean on popular opinion rather than seeking God for personal revelation and understanding regarding their health choices. Just because some individuals claim that using medicine is a lack of faith does not make it true. Remember, our faith journey is personal, and we must seek God for guidance in all matters, including health.

Biblical Examples of Medical Interventions

The Bible contains numerous examples that show medical interventions are not contrary to God's will. Luke, the beloved physician, was one of Paul's close companions and a significant contributor to the New Testament (Colossians 4:14). If medical practice were against God's will, it is unlikely that Luke, a physician, would have been so highly regarded in the early church.

Additionally, Paul advised Timothy to take a little wine for his stomach's sake and his frequent ailments (1 Timothy 5:23). In this context, wine was used for medicinal purposes. This shows that even in the early church, there was an understanding and acceptance of using natural remedies to treat physical conditions.

If God approved the use of medicine in biblical times, why would He disapprove of it now? God does not change (Malachi 3:6), and His principles remain the same. He provides us with medical knowledge as part of His care for us, and we should not dismiss these resources out of a misguided sense of spirituality or faith.

Avoiding Extremes in Belief

It's important to avoid extremes when it comes to our beliefs about medicine and divine healing. While it's true that our ultimate trust should be in God, it doesn't mean we should disregard the tools He has given us. The enemy would like nothing more than to see believers suffer needlessly because of a lack of knowledge or because they have been misled by well-meaning but misguided teachings.

Hosea 4:6 says, **"*My people are destroyed for lack of knowledge.*"** It is critical that we educate ourselves about health and healing, both from a biblical perspective and through the knowledge God has provided to humanity through science and medicine. We should not view the two as opposing forces but as complementary aspects of God's provision for His people.

Moving Toward Divine Health

As you continue on your journey towards divine health, remember that medicine is not your enemy. Rather, it is a resource that God has provided to help you maintain your health as you build your faith in Him not to need them again.

It is not a substitute for faith, but it can work alongside your faith. Seek God's guidance in every decision you make regarding your health. Pray for wisdom, and don't be afraid to use the tools and resources available to you, including medicine.

Let your beliefs be grounded in God's Word and your personal revelation of His will for your life. As you grow in faith, continue to trust God as your ultimate healer while using the wisdom He provides to make informed decisions about your health. Remember, medicine and faith are not in opposition; they can work together to bring about the fullness of God's promise of divine health in your life. **If medical interventions were evil, it would be right to label doctors, pharmacists, and every other medical professional as 'devils'.**

"He himself bore our sins in his body on the tree, that we might die to sin and live to righteousness. By his wounds you have been healed." 1 Pet. 2:24

The same sacrifice for your sin settled your healing.

Chapter 3

My Testimony

Except for a few childhood health issues, I lived a completely sickness-free life until I was 17. However, after relocating to a new region, I suddenly became prone to illness and spent many weeks hospitalized over the course of a year. During this time, I was given various treatments—both medical and orthodox, including concoctions and herbal remedies. People around me were concerned for my well-being and offered a lot of advice—some godly and some ungodly.

Eventually, after we relocated again, my health stabilized. After I rededicated my life to Christ in 2008, I learned about divine health through Kenneth Hagin's books. I began to understand that divine health is not about denying the existence of sickness but about overcoming it through the knowledge of what Christ has already accomplished for us (1 Peter 2:24). This was a pivotal moment in my journey toward living in divine health. I believed, built, and released my faith in it.

Building Faith in Divine Health

During this time, the devil tested my faith. There were moments when I couldn't bear the pain, and I would turn to the dispensary for drugs. But even while taking the medicines, I would remind myself that living in divine health is feasible for me. I just needed to build my faith more and get it right the next time. As I grew in my understanding, I realized that medicine is not evil (John 3:27), and taking medication was not a sin. It was simply a means to sustain life while I built my faith.

To the glory of God, my story has changed! Some time ago, I visited the hospital for a comprehensive health check, and the doctor was amazed at my health, noting that my *Salmonella paratyphi* titre level was extremely high, yet I looked perfectly fine (*Salmonella Typhi* and *Salmonella Paratyphi* A are human-restricted organisms that cause typhoid fever.) I chuckled because I no longer operate under the world's principles. A greater law was engaged that suspended the natural laws—the law of the Spirit of life in Christ Jesus (Romans 8:2). To the glory of God, those titer levels have been long destroyed, and I now have a clean bill of health medically.

Growing in Faith Through Trials

Have I used drugs since understanding divine health? Yes. There were times when I was too busy and failed to nourish my faith, causing my health to succumb. In those moments, I realized my faith was low, so I took medication while diligently feeding my spirit with the Word of God. This reinforced my understanding that while we live in this world, our bodies are not yet fully redeemed and are still vulnerable to attacks. However, what we choose to believe and feed on determines the outcome.

Today, by God's grace, I can boldly say, "I cannot be sick!" This doesn't mean my body isn't sometimes attacked, but what's more real to me is the knowledge of what Jesus has done for my health. I remember once saying, "It wouldn't be fair to Jesus if, after all He's done for my health, I still got sick!" That wasn't just my mind speaking; it was my spirit, fully convinced of the truth of God's Word. This can be your testimony too! Everything concerning your health was settled at Calvary. Your understanding of this truth is your key to enjoying divine health. As we have discussed in the previous chapters, divine health is about aligning your beliefs with God's Word and taking practical steps to build your faith. This journey is personal and requires a continual feeding on God's Word and renewing your mind (Romans 12:2).

The Root of Many Health Issues: A Wrong Mindset

One of the biggest obstacles to living in divine health is a wrong mindset. I once heard a woman on the radio explaining how misconceptions about the body lead to unnecessary fear. She said many Africans mistakenly believe that any slight discoloration in their urine means they're sick, prompting them to take herbal concoctions. Often, the discoloration is simply due to dehydration, and what's needed is hydration therapy. By drinking an herbal mixture, which is usually water-based, they unknowingly rehydrate and attribute the change in urine color to the medicine working.

This struck a chord with me deeply. I realized how often our fears and misconceptions about health are based on incomplete or incorrect information. Later, I read in Papa Oyedepo's book, <u>Keys to Divine Health</u>, that urine discoloration doesn't necessarily indicate illness. But because of what I had been taught, I would get scared whenever I observed discoloration in my urine, thereby becoming a slave to fear.

When you believe that every mosquito bite leads to malaria, every irritation from any insect bite will make you think you have malaria. Proverbs 23:7 says, ***"For as he thinks in his heart, so is he."*** Our thoughts and beliefs have a powerful impact on our health. A wrong mindset opens the door to fear, and fear is one of the devil's greatest tools to rob us of the peace and confidence we have in Christ.

Changing Your Mindset

The key to overcoming this fear and living in divine health is to renew your mind with the Word of God. Romans 12:2 reminds us to be transformed by the renewing of our minds. We must replace our fear-based thinking with faith-based thinking. Faith comes by hearing, and hearing by the Word of God (Romans 10:17). As you immerse yourself in the truth of God's Word, your mindset will change, and you will begin to see yourself as God sees you—healthy, whole, and victorious.

Understanding the root of health issues is crucial to overcoming them. Many times, the root is not in the body but in the mind. Our bodies respond to what our minds believe. If we believe that sickness is inevitable or that every symptom is a sign of a serious disease, our bodies will respond accordingly. But if we believe in the finished work of Christ and that we were not created to be sick, our bodies will also respond accordingly.

Preparing for the Seven Keys

As we prepare to delve into the seven keys to divine health, I want to encourage you to open your heart to the truth of God's Word. The foundation we have laid so far is crucial to understanding and applying these keys. They are not just principles; they are life-changing truths that, when applied, can transform your health and your life. I believe that as you read and meditate on these truths, your life will never be the same again.

"He himself bore our sins in his body on the tree, that we might die to sin and live to righteousness. By his wounds you have been healed." 1 Pet. 2:24

The same sacrifice for your sin settled your healing.

Chapter 4

Key #1: Believe It!

The first key to living in divine health is believing that it is possible. You must accept and fully embrace the truth that you can live a sickness-free life. The Bible is clear: **"*For assuredly, I say to you, whoever says to this mountain, 'Be removed and be cast into the sea,' and does not doubt in his heart, but believes that those things he says will be done, he will have whatever he says*"** (Mark 11:23-24). Faith is the foundation for receiving anything from God, including divine health.

The Power of Belief

Belief is a powerful force. Many people experience relief from pain and sickness after taking certain medications not necessarily because those medicines have therapeutic properties, but because they believe they'll be relieved after taking them. This phenomenon is called the "placebo effect." It demonstrates how a person's belief can trigger real physical responses in the body, even when the treatment itself is inactive.

Let me explain with a story

In the 1970s, at St. Murumba's College, Jos, Nigeria, a group of second-year students were playing during a break. One of their friends appeared disinterested and looked unwell.

Concerned, the others asked him what was wrong, and he replied that he had a headache. One of his friends rushed to the next class, took a piece of chalk, carved it into tablet-sized pieces with a blade, and gave it to the "sick" boy, who took the "medicine" without any doubt.

A short while later, the boy joined the rest of the group in their play, appearing perfectly fine. The friend who gave him the "medicine" later revealed it was just chalk, accusing him of faking the headache. However, the boy insisted that the "medicine" had indeed relieved his headache. This was a clear example of the placebo effect in action. The boy's belief in the "medicine" was so strong that it actually alleviated his symptoms.

Believing Before Seeing

The lesson here is simple: You must first believe before you can see. Just as the boy believed he would be relieved after taking what he thought was medicine, you must believe it is possible to live in divine health. The Bible tells us, ***"By His stripes, you were healed"*** (1 Peter 2:24). Notice it says "were healed," not "will be healed." This means your healing was already accomplished over 2,000 years ago when Jesus took those stripes.

Many believers struggle with this because, while they have accepted Jesus as their Lord and Savior, they haven't fully grasped that Jesus is also their Healer. God declared Himself as Jehovah Rapha, "the Lord who heals you" (Exodus 15:26). Healing is a fundamental part of the salvation package. The

Greek word for salvation, *soteria*, encompasses healing, preservation, and soundness. You must believe in this all-encompassing provision to experience it fully.

Faith Comes by Hearing

Believing in divine health often requires renewing your mind and building your faith through the Word of God. Romans 10:17 says, ***"Faith comes by hearing, and hearing by the Word of God."*** It's not enough to hear it once; you need to immerse yourself in the Word continually. When Dr. Chris Oyakhilome first caught the revelation of divine healing, he often found himself in the hospital. Yet, he chose to believe it was real and persisted in his faith. Today, his story is different—he walks in divine health. Hallelujah!

Belief Beyond Understanding

It's important to note that just because you can't see something doesn't mean it doesn't exist. Take radio waves, for example. You can't see them, but when you dial a number on your phone, you believe someone will answer on the other end. Even if you don't fully understand how it all works, your belief enables you to benefit from it. Similarly, you don't need to understand all the mechanics of divine health to believe in it and experience it. Your faith is the key that unlocks this reality.

Lay Hold of Your Healing

To live in divine health, you must first believe it is possible. You must reject the mindset that sickness is inevitable and instead embrace the truth of God's Word. Just as we have fathers in the faith who have gone decades without being sick, this provision is available for every child of God—not just pastors or special ministers. As you continue to build your faith, remember that divine health is not just a possibility; it is your inheritance as a believer. Claim it, walk in it, and let the reality of what Jesus has done for you transform your health and life.

In the following chapters, we will explore additional keys to divine health. As you continue reading, let your heart be open, and allow your faith to grow. Remember, *all things are possible to those who believe* (Mark 9:23).

"He himself bore our sins in his body on the tree, that we might die to sin and live to righteousness. By his wounds you have been healed." 1 Pet. 2:24

The same sacrifice for your sin settled your healing.

Chapter 5

Key #2: Desire It

The second key to living in divine health is desire. Desire is not just a simple wish or fleeting thought; it is a deep, compelling force within you. It's the inner drive that compels you to pursue what you truly want. Desire is a powerful spiritual principle that attracts things into your life. Jesus said, "***Therefore I say to you, whatever things you desire when you pray, believe that you receive them, and you will have them***" (Mark 11:24). This scripture underscores the connection between desire, faith, and manifestation.

The Power of Desire

Desire is like a magnet; it pulls what you long for toward you. This concept is evident throughout the Bible. When you have a strong desire for something, it sets spiritual laws into motion, drawing that thing into your reality. In the story of the Tower of Babel (Genesis 11:1-9), the people had a unified desire to build a city and a tower that reached the heavens. Even though their motive was misguided, their strong desire and unity of purpose caused God to intervene directly to thwart their plans. That's the power of desire—it attracts forces, good or bad, to make things happen.

When you desire to live in perfect divine health, that desire becomes a spiritual force working on your behalf. It energizes you to pursue divine health with tenacity, even when you encounter obstacles or setbacks. Desire is what fuels your determination to see the promises of God manifest in your life, regardless of what your circumstances may currently look like.

Desire in the Bible

The Bible is filled with examples of individuals whose desires led them to miraculous outcomes. Take the woman with the issue of blood in Mark 5:25-34. She had suffered for twelve years, spending all she had on physicians without any improvement. Yet, her desire to be healed was so strong that she pressed through the crowd just to touch the hem of Jesus' garment. She said to herself, ***"If I may touch but His clothes, I shall be whole"*** (Mark 5:28). Her desire, coupled with faith, activated the power of God, and she was instantly healed.

Similarly, blind Bartimaeus in Mark 10:46-52 had a burning desire to see. When he heard that Jesus was passing by, he cried out, ***"Jesus, Son of David, have mercy on me!"*** Even when people around him told him to be quiet, his desire pushed him to cry out even louder. Jesus responded to his persistent desire and healed him. ***"What do you want Me to do for you?" Jesus asked. Bartimaeus replied, "Rabboni, that I may receive my sight." And Jesus said to him, "Go your way; your faith has made you well." Immediately, he received his sight and followed Jesus on the road.***

Desire Aligns with God's Will

Desiring divine health is in alignment with God's will for your life. God's Word declares in 3 John 1:2, **_Beloved, I pray that you may prosper in all things and be in health, just as your soul prospers._** God wants you to be healthy. When your desires align with His will, you position yourself to receive His blessings. Desire is the starting point of all achievement, and when your desire is focused on divine health, it releases God's healing power into your life.

Desire also drives you to take practical steps toward achieving divine health. It may prompt you to immerse yourself in God's Word, build your faith, and develop a prayer life that aligns with God's promises. Desire motivates you to feed your spirit with teachings that reinforce the truth about divine health, like reading books, listening to sermons, or sharing testimonies that build faith. It creates an internal hunger for the things of God, which in turn, fosters spiritual growth and a deeper understanding of His will for your life.

The Right Kind of Desire

Not all desires are beneficial. The Bible warns about desires that lead to sin and destruction. James 1:14-15 says, **_But each one is tempted when he is drawn away by his own desires and enticed. Then, when desire has conceived, it gives birth to sin; and sin, when it is full-grown, brings forth death._** Therefore, it is crucial to ensure that your desires are in line with God's Word. A godly desire for divine health is not just about being free from sickness; it is about living a life that glorifies God in your body and spirit, which are His (1 Corinthians 6:19-20).

Stirring Up Your Desire for Divine Health

To see divine health become a reality in your life, you must cultivate and maintain a strong desire for it. This means regularly renewing your mind with God's promises about health and healing. Speak God's Word over your life daily, affirming your desire to walk in divine health. Surround yourself with people and resources that encourage and support your desire. Remember, when your desire is right and strong enough, it will pull the necessary spiritual forces in your direction to make things happen.

Desire also keeps you motivated, even when you haven't yet seen the results you want. It propels you to keep pressing forward, trusting in God's Word and His promises, no matter what. The woman with the issue of blood didn't give up after twelve years of suffering. Blind Bartimaeus didn't keep silent when others tried to quiet him. They both had a strong, unwavering desire that fueled their faith and led to their miraculous healing.

Cultivate Your Desire

Desire is a divine force that God has placed in every human being to accomplish great things. When your desire is aligned with God's will, it becomes a powerful tool that attracts the promises of God into your life. If you desire to live in divine health, let that desire be strong and unwavering. **Pray about** it, speak it, and take steps toward it. As you do, you will see the manifestation of God's healing power in your life, and divine health will become your reality.

"He himself bore our sins in his body on the tree, that we might die to sin and live to righteousness. By his wounds you have been healed." 1 Pet. 2:24

The same sacrifice for your sin settled your healing.

Chapter 6
Key #3: Despise Sickness

The third key to living in divine health is to despise sickness. This may seem like a strong statement, but it is a necessary mindset for anyone who desires to live a life free from sickness and disease. You cannot despise something and desire it at the same time. To live in divine health, you must both desire a sickness-free life and despise sickness itself.

The Power of Despising

Despising something means having a deep-seated aversion or repulsion to it. It's more than just disliking it—it's an intense rejection of its presence or influence in your life. In the same way that desire attracts what you want, despising something pushes it away from you. You need to understand that if the force of desire attracts, the force of despise repels. Just as nature abhors a vacuum, you must fill the space of your mind and life with health and vitality so that sickness cannot find room to enter.

To despise sickness means to reject it with all your being, to see it as something foreign and unwanted. Some people, however, have unknowingly cultivated an attachment to sickness. They secretly admire the attention they receive when they are unwell. They enjoy having people come to visit and care for them, treating sickness almost like a beloved guest rather than a hostile intruder. They have even gone so far as to personalize their conditions, saying things like "my high blood pressure" or "my arthritis," claiming ownership over what they should be rejecting.

Stop Glorifying Sickness

The moment you decide to despise sickness, you will no longer glorify it by talking about it or claiming it as your own. You will no longer say things like "my flu" or "my diabetes." Instead, you will speak words of life and health. Even when your body is challenged, you will not make a spectacle of it or seek sympathy from others. You will simply acknowledge that your body needs rest to recuperate, rather than blowing trumpets and drawing attention to a condition that Jesus has already taken away.

It is essential to have the same attitude towards sickness as you do towards sin. Just as you despise and reject sin because Jesus took it away on the cross, you must also despise and reject sickness. Imagine sickness as a waste product you have no interest in associating with. Jesus took your sins and your sicknesses; you don't need them, and you should not accept them!

Rejecting Sickness as an Unwanted Guest

Think of sickness as an unwelcome guest trying to enter your home. If a thief or a harmful person were at your door, you wouldn't invite them in and make them comfortable—you would lock the door and call for help. In the same way, when symptoms of sickness try to enter your life, you must refuse to entertain them. Speak against them with the authority given to you by Jesus. Remember what Jesus said in John 10:10, *"The thief comes only to steal and kill and destroy; I have come that they may have life, and have it to the full."* Sickness is a thief, and Jesus has already provided a way for you to live a full, abundant life free from it.

Stand Firm in the Victory of Jesus

The Bible tells us that Jesus bore our sicknesses and carried our pains (Isaiah 53:4-5). This means that every sickness and disease was already dealt with at the cross. Why, then, would you want to hold onto something that Jesus has taken away? It would be like clinging to your old sinful habits even after being saved. Instead, you must despise sickness in the same way you despise sin and stand firm in the victory that Jesus has won for you.

Galatians 3:13 says, *"Christ redeemed us from the curse of the law by becoming a curse for us."* Sickness is part of the curse of the law, but Jesus has redeemed you from it. Knowing this, you should be bold in your stand against sickness. Do not allow it to remain in your life for a moment longer than necessary. Speak to it, command it to leave, and believe that God's promise of health and healing is true for you today.

Think of sickness as an unwelcome guest trying to enter your home. If a thief or a harmful person were at your door, you wouldn't invite them in and make them comfortable—you would lock the door and call for help. In the same way, when symptoms of sickness try to enter your life, you must refuse to entertain them. Speak against them with the authority given to you by Jesus. Remember what Jesus said in John 10:10, *"The thief comes only to steal and kill and destroy; I have come that they may have life, and have it to the full."* Sickness is a thief, and Jesus has already provided a way for you to live a full, abundant life free from it.

Stand Firm in the Victory of Jesus

The Bible tells us that Jesus bore our sicknesses and carried our pains (Isaiah 53:4-5). This means that every sickness and disease was already dealt with at the cross. Why, then, would you want to hold onto something that Jesus has taken away? It would be like clinging to your old sinful habits even after being saved. Instead, you must despise sickness in the same way you despise sin and stand firm in the victory that Jesus has won for you.

Galatians 3:13 says, *"Christ redeemed us from the curse of the law by becoming a curse for us."* Sickness is part of the curse of the law, but Jesus has redeemed you from it. Knowing this, you should be bold in your stand against sickness. Do not allow it to remain in your life for a moment longer than necessary. Speak to it, command it to leave, and believe that God's promise of health and healing is true for you today.

You Don't Need What Jesus Took Away

To despise sickness is to see it for what it truly is: a defeated enemy. Sickness is not something to be coddled or accepted; it is something to be cast out and rejected. Jesus has already borne the burden of your sickness and pain so that you do not have to. When you truly grasp this, you will begin to see sickness as a waste product—something you are not willing to associate with or accept in any form.

Remember, Jesus took your sicknesses, and you don't need them. Reject them with all your might, despise them as you despise sin, and walk in the freedom and health that God has provided for you. As you continue to apply this key to your life, you will see the power of God's Word manifest in your health, and you will live in the divine health that is rightfully yours in Christ Jesus. Hallelujah!

"He himself bore our sins in his body on the tree, that we might die to sin and live to righteousness. By his wounds you have been healed." 1 Pet. 2:24

The same sacrifice for your sin settled your healing.

Chapter 7

Key #4: Think Health

The fourth key to living in divine health is to think health. The Bible teaches us the importance of our thoughts and the impact they have on our lives. Proverbs 4:23 says, **"Keep thy heart with all diligence; for out of it are the issues of life."** This verse highlights that our hearts and minds are the source of all the issues we face in life, including our health. The thoughts you entertain in your mind form pictures that shape your beliefs, and those beliefs dictate what you say and ultimately what you experience in your life.

The Power of Thought

Your thought life is a powerful tool that can either bring you health or sickness. Jesus said in Matthew 12:34, **"For out of the abundance of the heart, the mouth speaketh."** Your thoughts fill your heart, and your mouth eventually speaks what is in your heart. And according to the power of creation, as described in the Bible, you are permitted to have what you say. Mark 11:23 reinforces this truth: **"For verily I say unto you, That whosoever shall say unto this mountain, Be thou removed, and be thou cast into the sea; and shall not doubt in his heart, but shall believe that those things which he saith shall come to pass; he shall have whatsoever he saith."** If your thoughts are filled with sickness, your mouth will inevitably speak words that align with sickness, and your body will respond to those words. You cannot think of sickness and live a healthy life. It is crucial to align your thoughts with health, vitality, and divine healing. Your thoughts shape your words, and your words shape your life!

Think About These Things

To think healthily, you must train your mind to dwell on thoughts that promote life and healing. Philippians 4:8 provides a powerful benchmark for your thoughts: ***"Finally, brethren, whatsoever things are true, whatsoever things are honest, whatsoever things are just, whatsoever things are pure, whatsoever things are lovely, whatsoever things are of good report; if there be any virtue, and if there be any praise, think on these things."*** If a thought fails to meet the criteria set in this scripture, it must be dealt with in the name of Jesus. Your thought life remains a viable channel into your life; therefore, you must guard it diligently!

Every thought that does not align with divine health should be taken captive and made obedient to Christ, as Paul instructs in 2 Corinthians 10:5: ***"Casting down imaginations, and every high thing that exalteth itself against the knowledge of God, and bringing into captivity every thought to the obedience of Christ."*** When a thought of sickness enters your mind, you must counterattack it with a scripture from God's Word about your health. Speak life over yourself, and do not allow any room for thoughts of sickness or disease to take root. Constantly plead the blood of Jesus against such thoughts.

Thoughts Are Seeds

Consider your thoughts as seeds. When you plant seeds in a garden, they eventually grow and bear fruit. In the same way, the thoughts you plant in your mind will grow and bear fruit in your life. If you plant thoughts of sickness, fear, and anxiety, you will harvest sickness, fear, and anxiety. But if you plant thoughts of health, peace, and divine healing, you will harvest health, peace, and healing.

Jesus said in Luke 6:45, **_A good man out of the good treasure of his heart bringeth forth that which is good; and an evil man out of the evil treasure of his heart bringeth forth that which is evil: for of the abundance of the heart his mouth speaketh._** Your heart is the soil, and your thoughts are the seeds. Make sure you are planting good seeds that will bring forth a good harvest in your life.

The Battle for the Mind

In my own life, I have noticed that each time the devil successfully steals from me, he first gains access to my mind. When the enemy wants to bring sickness into your life, he often starts by firing a thought of sickness into your mind. It might be a fleeting thought of "What if I get sick?" or "I'm feeling a bit under the weather." If you entertain these thoughts, they can grow into fear and eventually manifest in your body.

However, you have the authority to counter these thoughts with the Word of God. Whenever a thought of sickness is fired into your mind, immediately counterattack it with a scripture about your health and healing. For example, declare Isaiah 53:5, ***"But he was wounded for our transgressions, he was bruised for our iniquities: the chastisement of our peace was upon him; and with his stripes, we are healed."*** By speaking the Word of God over your life, you are planting seeds of health and divine healing that will produce a harvest of health in your body. Joyce Meyer dealt with this in her book, "The Battle Field of the Mind". I strongly recommend it.

Guard Your Mind

To live in divine health, you must think about health. Your mind is a battlefield, and you must guard it with all diligence. Do not allow thoughts of sickness, disease, or fear to take root in your mind. Instead, fill your mind with the Word of God and thoughts that promote health, life, and peace. Remember, ***"As a man thinketh in his heart, so is he"*** (Proverbs 23:7). Your thoughts have the power to shape your reality, so choose to think healthily and live a life free from sickness and disease.

As you continue to align your thoughts with the truth of God's Word, you will see the manifestation of divine health in your life. Your mind is a powerful tool that God has given you to create the life you desire. Use it wisely, think healthily, and experience the fullness of the abundant life that Jesus came to give you. Hallelujah!

"He himself bore our sins in his body on the tree, that we might die to sin and live to righteousness. By his wounds you have been healed." 1 Pet. 2:24

The same sacrifice for your sin settled your healing.

Chapter 8

Key #5: Use Your Drugs

The fifth key to living in divine health is to use your drugs. But here, we're not talking about conventional medicine. The Bible refers to the Word of God as medicine: *"My son, attend to my words; incline thine ear unto my sayings. Let them not depart from thine eyes; keep them in the midst of thine heart. For they are life unto those that find them, and health to all their flesh"* (Proverbs 4:20-22). Just as we take medicine to prevent or cure illness, we should also take the Word of God as medicine for our bodies and souls.

Two Approaches to Drug Administration

In pharmacology, there are two main approaches to administering drugs:

- Prophylactic/Preventive: This approach focuses on preventing illness before it occurs. Vaccinations are a prime example; they build up the immune system to combat specific pathogens. However, they are not universal—no single vaccine can prevent all diseases.
- Curative: This approach treats illnesses after they have occurred.

Similarly, the Word of God can be used both as a preventive measure or a cure. The best approach, however, is to take it preventively, building your spiritual and physical immunity before sickness strikes.

How to Take the Word of God as Medicine

Locate Scriptures on Health: The Bible is filled with scriptures that speak about healing, health, and wholeness. It is crucial to search for these verses and make them a part of your daily life. You can use a Bible search engine or refer to books that compile healing scriptures. One such book is "ARISE AND BE HEALED" by Faith Oyedepo, who used these scriptures when faced with a personal health challenge.

Recite Them Daily to Yourself: Our bodies are designed with two ears—the outer ear and the inner ear. The inner ear is uniquely connected to your spirit and picks up the vibrations of your voice more powerfully than any external sound. This is why your own voice sounds different to you when played back on a recording. Speaking healing scriptures aloud to yourself allows your spirit to hear these affirmations directly, reinforcing your belief in them. Remember, everything God has made, including your body, is sustained by His Word (Hebrews 1:3). This is a Do-It-Yourself (DIY) process that God has set for us; He won't do it for you. Make it a habit to speak health over your body daily, even when you are not sick.

Testimony of Faith in Action

A friend of mine, Femi Ibidunmoye, shared a story about his mother who faced a mysterious health challenge. Doctors were unable to diagnose the cause, so she was sent home without a cure. Femi began to recite two healing scriptures with her every morning and evening, just as one would take prescribed medication. Initially, he saw no change and felt discouraged, but his mother insisted they continue because she felt relieved each time they spoke the scriptures. They resumed the routine, and over time, she was miraculously healed. This story illustrates the power of consistently applying God's Word as medicine.

You don't have to see it to believe it. Start declaring your healing now. For instance, I daily declare, "I have been healed by the stripes of Christ over two thousand years ago, so, therefore, I cannot be sick." I also say, "I am an inhabitant of Zion, therefore, it shall never be heard of me that I am sick!" I apply this principle not only to my health but to every area of my life. Don't wait until sickness comes before you start doing this. Make it a daily routine.

Another Example: I confess strength every day. You will never hear me say, "I am tired," regardless of how I feel. At most, I might say, "My body needs rest." Words matter! The Bible says, ***"Let the weak say I am strong"*** (Joel 3:10)

How the Word of God Operates

The Word of God operates systemically, from the inside out. This is similar to how certain herbicides work. There are contact herbicides that kill weeds from the point of contact and systemic herbicides that get absorbed into the plant's system, travel to the roots and kill it from there. The systemic herbicides take longer to show visible results, but their effects are more profound and long-lasting. Similarly, the Word of God might not show immediate visible effects, but it works deep within us, and its impact becomes evident over time. You must believe in its power and keep applying it consistently.

Speak to Your Body

Speaking to your body is crucial for maintaining divine health. The moment you speak, something happens within you. A Japanese scientist, Masaru Emoto, conducted a study on the power of words and their effect on objects. He placed cooked white rice in two jars labeled "Thank you" and "You fool," and had primary school students read these labels aloud twice daily. After 30 days, the rice in the "You fool" jar had turned into a black gelatinous mass, while the rice in the "Thank you" jar remained fresh. This experiment demonstrates the profound impact of words.

Furthermore, Emoto also researched the effects of words on water. He concluded that speaking to water induces radioactivity. Considering that at least 70% of the human body is water, your words can significantly affect your physical health. To live in perfect divine health, you must learn to speak positive words over your body consistently. Say things like, "My body is strong and healthy," "I am full of energy and vitality," or "I am free from sickness and disease." Your words carry power; use them wisely to maintain your health.

Consistent Application is Key

Using the Word of God as medicine involves consistently speaking and believing in its power to heal and maintain your health. It's about building a strong foundation that prevents sickness and promotes divine health. Just as you wouldn't wait until you're sick to start taking preventive medicine, don't wait until a health challenge arises before you start applying God's Word. Make it a daily practice, and you will see the manifestation of divine health in your life. Remember, **"The word of God is quick, and powerful, and sharper than any two-edged sword"** (Hebrews 4:12). Use it daily, and experience the fullness of health and vitality that God has promised. Hallelujah!

"He himself bore our sins in his body on the tree, that we might die to sin and live to righteousness. By his wounds you have been healed." 1 Pet. 2:24

The same sacrifice for your sin settled your healing.

Chapter 9
Key #6: Obey the Laws

The sixth key to living in divine health is to obey the laws. Life is governed by laws, both natural and spiritual, and these laws are designed to safeguard our lives. If you desire to live a long and healthy life, it is crucial to understand and obey these laws. Laws must not be ignored or abused; instead, they should be respected and followed diligently.

Laws exist to protect us, and breaking them often comes with consequences. However, if you must break one law, you must be operating under a higher law that suspends the effect of the other. For example, the law of gravity is a universal law that pulls objects downward. It is not affected by one's age, race, or beliefs. But the laws of thrust and lift, which govern flight, can suspend gravity. Airplanes operate by these twin laws to overcome gravity's pull. Similarly, there are laws for life that relate to our health and well-being. Let's explore some of these laws that are essential for maintaining divine health.

1. The Law of Rest

The first law for maintaining good health is the law of rest. To live a sound and vibrant life, you must obey this law. Rest is not just a suggestion; it is a divine mandate. While God was creating the earth and everything in it, He instituted the law of rest by taking time off from His work on the seventh day (Genesis 2:2-3). This action was not due to fatigue or weariness—God, who is all-powerful, never grows tired. Instead, it was to set an example for us, highlighting the importance of rest in the earth realm. This goes to show that among the several attributes of this earth realm is rest. Notice that after the creation of the earth, there has been no mention of God resting again. This underscores that rest is particularly important in our earthly existence.

Rest is more than just physical sleep; it is a state of mental, emotional, and spiritual rejuvenation. Pastor E. A. Adeboye describes rest as doing the exact opposite of what you have been doing for a long time. If you have been sitting for hours, rest means standing up and taking a walk. If you have been engaged in mentally strenuous activities, rest could mean engaging in something relaxing and refreshing. Incorporating periods of rest into your daily routine is essential to rejuvenate your mind, body, and spirit.

The importance of rest cannot be overemphasized. Many people today are overworked, stressed, and burnt out because they neglect this vital principle. Rest is a necessary component of divine health, and it should not be ignored. To experience the fullness of health God intends for us, we must learn to rest properly and regularly.

2. Eat Well

The second law is to eat well. After creating man, God immediately gave him instructions on what to eat (Genesis 1:29). If food were not important, God would not have emphasized it. Just like a car manufacturer specifies the type of fuel a car should run on, God, who created us, knows what we need to remain functional and healthy on earth. Don't neglect the importance of food. This is not to promote gluttony but rather to emphasize the importance of eating wisely and appropriately.

An adage says, "When you eat your food as medicine, you won't need to take your medicine as food." I can personally relate to this as I used to have a very poor eating habit, not because of lack, but due to my own beliefs and practices. I have since learned the importance of eating well.

How to Feed Yourself

Man is a triune being—spirit, soul, and body (1 Thessalonians 5:23). To maintain a healthy and vibrant life, you must feed all three parts adequately:

COMPARTMENT	FOOD
Spirit	The Word of God through prints, audio, or visual
Soul	Inspirational books, music and movies
Body	Natural foods

However, it is essential to prioritize feeding your spirit and soul, as these have eternal value.

3. Live Right

The third law is to live right. This involves practicing good hygiene and making healthy lifestyle choices. The Lord once laid it on my heart to always wash my hands whenever I come home from an outing, and to brush my teeth before going to bed. God's instructions are for our good, not His. Many infectious diseases, like salmonellosis, are transmitted through contaminated food and water. As we go about our daily activities, we come into contact with various surfaces that may harbor germs. It is crucial to wash your hands regularly, especially before eating. Better still, have a bath to cleanse your body of impurities.

Similarly, maintaining oral hygiene is essential. My mother suffered from dental problems when I was younger, which may be why God emphasized this practice to me. Simple acts like these can prevent many health problems. For instance, the Bible does not explicitly say, "Do not smoke," but it does instruct us to honor our bodies, which are temples of God (1 Corinthians 3:16-17). Medical experts warn that smoking damages the lungs, a vital part of our body. Obeying these simple laws will protect your health.

I recall a friend who once used a skin cream that caused severe burns and left a permanent scar on her face. Many people, in their quest for beauty, have ended up damaging their skin and contracting illnesses such as skin cancer from harmful beauty products. This underscores the importance of living right and making informed choices.

The Benefits of Obeying God's Laws

Obeying God's laws and principles, as well as sound medical advice (as long as it does not contradict God's Word), will keep us safe and healthy. God's commandments are designed for our benefit, and they encompass all aspects of our lives, including our health. Remember, the laws of God and the wisdom in His Word are meant to protect us and help us live full, vibrant lives. By obeying these laws—resting, eating well, and living right—you position yourself to enjoy the fullness of life God has planned for you. Embrace these laws, and experience divine health and longevity. Hallelujah!

"He himself bore our sins in his body on the tree, that we might die to sin and live to righteousness. By his wounds you have been healed." 1 Pet. 2:24

The same sacrifice for your sin settled your healing.

Chapter 10

Key #7: Ownership

The seventh key to living in divine health is understanding the concept of ownership. Ownership is a powerful principle. No genuine owner of anything valuable will watch it waste away without doing something about it. A true owner will guard their possessions jealously to ensure they are kept safe and sound. When you own something, you take responsibility for it, nurture it, and protect it from harm. This principle applies to our health and well-being as well.

Reasons Why People Own Things

There are several reasons why people take ownership of things:

- **Purpose**: People often own things because they serve a specific purpose. For example, a carpenter owns tools that are essential for his craft, and a student owns books to aid in learning. Ownership is tied to utility and function.
- **Prestige**: Ownership can also be a matter of prestige. People may own luxury items, such as cars or houses, as a symbol of their status or achievements. Ownership, in this sense, is linked to honor and recognition.

- **Pleasure Derived**: Lastly, people own things because of the pleasure they derive from them. It could be a favorite hobby, a cherished piece of art, or a beloved pet. Ownership here is about joy and satisfaction.

But the question is, who owns your body?

Accepting Jesus as your Lord and Savior makes Him the rightful owner of your body. The Bible makes it clear that once you give your life to Christ, you no longer belong to yourself. In 2 Corinthians 6:16, the Bible says, ***"For you are the temple of the living God."*** Similarly, in 1 Corinthians 3:19-20, it reminds us that God's Spirit dwells in us.

Why Does God Own Our Bodies?

- **Purpose**: God created us for a purpose. We are here to serve Him and fulfill His divine will. Genesis 1:26 states that God made man in His own image to have dominion over the earth. Revelation 4:11 also says that we were created for God's pleasure and to fulfill His purpose.
- **Prestige**: God takes pride in His children. Just as a parent delight in the achievements of their child, God delights in us. He loves to boast about us, as seen in Job 1:8, where God proudly mentions Job's righteousness to Satan. In Matthew 17:5, God expresses His pleasure in Jesus, saying, ***"This is my beloved Son, in whom I am well pleased."***

- **Pleasure**: God derives great pleasure from His creation. He finds joy in our worship, our obedience, and our relationship with Him. Matthew 5:16 encourages us to let our light shine so others may see our good deeds and glorify our Father in heaven.

God has done everything necessary to keep us healthy and whole. Psalm 107:20 says, ***"He sent His word and healed them and delivered them from their destructions."*** Likewise, 1 Peter 2:9 declares that we are a chosen generation, called to declare the praises of God. Our bodies, therefore, belong to Him.

The Illustration of Jesus Cleansing the Temple

Let me paint a picture for you: In the Bible, when Jesus entered the temple and saw people trading inside, He physically drove them out.

Why?

Because His Father's temple is not a place for rogues, but a house of prayer (Matthew 21:12-13). This incident is symbolic of our bodies. The moment Jesus comes into our lives, He begins to cleanse us from everything that defiles— every sickness, pain, and disease. Revelation 3:20 says, ***"Behold, I stand at the door and knock. If anyone hears my voice and opens the door, I will come in and eat with him, and he with me."*** When we allow God to own our bodies, He takes over the responsibility of keeping us safe and healthy. He drives out every spiritual "trader" causing harm to His temple, which is our body.

Has God Owned Your Body?

As I often say, God is everybody's Creator, but He is not the Father of every creature. Until you accept Jesus as your Lord and Savior, you remain a creature of God. Salvation grants you the privilege of a higher level of relationship with Him. He becomes your Father, and you become His child. With this relationship, He assumes full responsibility for your well-being. If you are an auto mechanic and your car has a problem, would you discard it, or would you fix it? Similarly, when God owns your life, He will begin to jealously guard everything that pertains to you.

No sane person would prioritize a stranger over their child if both are calling for attention at the same time. Matthew 7:11 puts it this way: ***"If you then, being evil, know how to give good gifts to your children, how much more shall your Father which is in heaven give good things to them that ask Him?"*** When God owns your body, He takes care of it with even greater diligence.

Practical Steps to Take Ownership of Your Body

1. Accept Jesus as Your Lord and Savior: The first step to letting God own your body is to accept Jesus into your life. This means acknowledging His sacrifice on the cross and receiving the gift of salvation. If you are ready to do this, please say this prayer:

"Lord Jesus, I receive You today as my Lord and Savior. I acknowledge the work You did on the cross for my sake, and I come to receive the free gift of salvation through faith. I declare that I no longer belong to the devil; I now belong to God through the words of my mouth. Thank You, Lord, for saving me. In Jesus' name, I pray. Amen."

If you have just said this prayer, congratulations! Your journey to health and wholeness begins here. I would love to hear your testimony; please email me at emmanuelanuoluwatomiwa@gmail.com. It is well with you in Jesus' name.

2. Live with the Consciousness of Divine Ownership: Understand that your body is now God's property, and treat it with respect and care. Avoid habits and lifestyles that could harm your body, and instead, engage in activities that promote physical, mental, and spiritual well-being.

3. Speak to Your Body with Authority: If you have given your life to Christ and the devil is afflicting your body, speak to it with the authority of a child of God. Philippians 2:9 reminds us that Jesus has been given a name above every name. Use this authority to command sickness, pain, and any affliction to leave your body in Jesus' name.

4. Maintain a Healthy Lifestyle: Honor God by taking good care of your body. Eat well, exercise regularly, rest, and maintain good hygiene. Remember, your body is the temple of the Holy Spirit, and it should be kept holy and healthy.

The Benefits of Letting God Own Your Body

When God owns your body, He takes responsibility for its health and well-being. He protects you, keeps you safe, and provides for all your needs. Just as a parent takes care of their child, God will take care of you. Make a conscious decision today to surrender your life and your body to Him. Trust Him to lead you into a life of divine health, peace, and fulfillment. Hallelujah!

"He himself bore our sins in his body on the tree, that we might die to sin and live to righteousness. By his wounds you have been healed." 1 Pet. 2:24

The same sacrifice for your sin settled your healing.

Chapter 11

Scriptural Confessions for Healing, Health, and Wholeness

As you journey towards living in divine health, it's important to understand that words have power. Proverbs 18:21 tells us that "death and life are in the power of the tongue." Therefore, speaking God's Word over your life daily is like taking a dose of medicine for your soul, spirit, and body. Here are some scriptural confessions to help you maintain your health, healing, and wholeness. Speak these words aloud in faith, believing that God's promises are true and that they will manifest in your life.

General Confessions for Healing and Health

1. **Confession for General Health:**

   "I declare that I am fearfully and wonderfully made. My body is a temple of the Holy Spirit, and I honor God with it (Psalm 139:14; 1 Corinthians 6:19-20). I am healthy, strong, and full of life. No sickness or disease can come near me, for the Lord is my healer and my protector (Exodus 15:26; Psalm 91:10)."

2. **Confession for Healing:**

   "I confess that by the stripes of Jesus, I am healed (Isaiah 53:5; 1 Peter 2:24). I refuse to allow sickness to have any place in my body.

Every cell, tissue, organ, and system of my body functions perfectly as God designed it to (Psalm 103:3). I speak life to my body and command it to align with God's Word in Jesus' name."

3. **Confession for Wholeness**:

"I am complete in Christ, who is the head over every power and authority (Colossians 2:10). I declare that I am whole—spirit, soul, and body. I have the mind of Christ, and I walk in divine wisdom and understanding (1 Corinthians 2:16; James 1:5)."

4. **Confession for Strength and Vitality**:

"The Lord is the strength of my life (Psalm 27:1). I can do all things through Christ who strengthens me (Philippians 4:13). My youth is renewed like the eagle's (Psalm 103:5). I am strong in the Lord and in the power of His might (Ephesians 6:10)."

Confessions for Specific Health Conditions

1. **Confession for Heart Health:**

"My heart is strong and healthy. The life of God flows through my veins, and His healing power is at work in every part of my cardiovascular system. I declare that my blood

pressure is normal, and my cholesterol levels
are balanced. I have a healthy heart because
God is the strength of my heart and my portion
forever (Psalm 73:26)."

2. **Confession for Diabetes**:

"I declare that my pancreas functions perfectly.
My body produces the right amount of insulin,
and my blood sugar levels are normal. I am free
from every form of diabetes, in Jesus' name. I
thank You, Lord, that You have blessed my
bread and water and taken sickness away from
me (Exodus 23:25)."

3. **Confession for Mental Health**:

"I have the mind of Christ, and I hold the
thoughts, feelings, and purposes of His heart (1
Corinthians 2:16). I declare that I have a sound
mind. I am free from fear, anxiety, depression,
and confusion. God has not given me a spirit of
fear, but of power, love, and a sound mind (2
Timothy 1:7). My mind is at peace, and my
thoughts are aligned with God's Word
(Philippians 4:8)."

4. **Confession for Digestive Health**:

"I declare that my digestive system functions
perfectly. My body absorbs all the nutrients it

needs, and I am free from any digestive disorders. Every part of my digestive system—from my mouth to my intestines—operates in perfect harmony, as God intended it to. I am healed and whole by the power of God (Matthew 15:13)."

5. **Confession for Respiratory Health:**

"I declare that my lungs are healthy and function perfectly. I am free from asthma, bronchitis, and any other respiratory conditions. The breath of God fills my lungs, and I breathe freely and deeply. The Lord is the breath of my life (Job 33:4)."

6. **Confession for Immune System Health:**

"I declare that my immune system is strong and healthy. It functions as God created it to, protecting my body from all sickness, disease, and infection. No weapon formed against me shall prosper (Isaiah 54:17). I am surrounded by a shield of God's favor, and I live in divine health (Psalm 5:12)."

7. **Confession for Joint and Bone Health:**

"I declare that my bones and joints are strong and healthy. My bones are not brittle, but they are filled with the strength and vitality of God.

The Lord renews my strength, and I walk
without pain or discomfort. I am free from
arthritis and any joint-related issues. The Word
of God is life to my bones and health to all my
flesh (Proverbs 4:20-22)."

8. **Confession for Cancer-Free Health**:

"I declare that my body is cancer-free. Every
abnormal cell in my body is removed and
replaced with healthy cells. The life of God
flows through my body, destroying every
cancerous cell and restoring perfect health. I am
fearfully and wonderfully made, and no disease
can take residence in my body. I am healed by
the power of Jesus' name (Philippians 2:9-10)."

9. **Confession for Reproductive Health**:

"I declare that my reproductive system is
healthy and functions perfectly. I am free from
any disorders, pain, or complications. I thank
God for blessing me with the ability to
conceive and carry children to full term. My
body is fruitful and flourishes according to
God's design (Genesis 1:28)."

10. **Confession for Skin Health**:

"I declare that my skin is healthy and radiant. I am
free from any skin conditions, including eczema,

psoriasis, acne, and rashes. My skin is a reflection of God's glory, and it is smooth, clear, and beautiful. I am fearfully and wonderfully made, and my skin is a testimony of God's handiwork (Psalm 139:14)."

Confessions for Emotional and Spiritual Wholeness

1. **Confession for Emotional Healing:**

   "I declare that I am free from all past hurts, rejection, and trauma. I choose to forgive those who have wronged me, and I release every offense. I am healed emotionally and made whole. The peace of God guards my heart and mind through Christ Jesus (Philippians 4:7)."

2. **Confession for Spiritual Strength:**

   "I declare that I am spiritually strong and mature. I feed on the Word of God daily, and my faith is growing exceedingly. I am led by the Spirit of God, and I walk in His wisdom and revelation (Ephesians 1:17). I am more than a conqueror through Him who loves me (Romans 8:37)."

3. **Confession for Overcoming Fear:**

   "I declare that I am free from all fear. God has not given me a spirit of fear, but of power, love, and a sound mind (2 Timothy 1:7). I am bold and courageous, for the Lord my God is with me wherever I go (Joshua 1:9)."

Final Confession for Daily Victory

"I declare that I live in divine health, healing, and wholeness every day of my life. I am strong in the Lord and in the power of His might. I walk in the fullness of God's promises, and I live a life that glorifies Him. No weapon formed against me shall prosper, and every tongue that rises against me in judgment I shall condemn (Isaiah 54:17). I am more than a conqueror through Christ who loves me, and I give all glory to God for my health, healing, and wholeness (Romans 8:37). Amen!"

These confessions are your spiritual medication for healing, health, and wholeness. Speak them daily, believe them, and watch as God's Word transforms your life. Remember, God's Word is life and health to all who find it. Stay blessed and live in divine health!

"He himself bore our sins in his body on the tree, that we might die to sin and live to righteousness. By his wounds you have been healed." 1 Pet. 2:24

The same sacrifice for your sin settled your healing.

Chapter 12

Conclusion

As we conclude this book, I believe that the power of God has touched and transformed you through the words shared in these pages. If you've noticed, after each chapter, I included a familiar verse:

"He Himself bore our sins in His body on the tree, that we might die to sin and live to righteousness. By His wounds you have been healed." 1 Peter 2:24.

The same sacrifice that dealt with your sin has also settled your healing.

I repeated this intentionally—it was for emphasis, so it could sink into your heart and spirit.

I remember an experience I had several years ago while living in Araga, Epe, Lagos. It was a Sunday morning, and I was on my way to church when I suddenly heard myself say, *"I wouldn't be fair to Jesus if I am still being sick."* At the time, I didn't fully understand the depth of that statement, but as the days passed, it became clearer.

Let me explain it this way: Imagine you owed a bank a significant loan, and the due date for payment had passed.

The bank's loan agents constantly harass you with calls and threats. You are so intimidated by their persistence that you stop answering unknown numbers and limit your movements to avoid any confrontation. Then, without your knowledge, a generous relative hears about your predicament and decides to pay off the entire loan.

When you discover the debt has been cleared, you realize that the harassment was unnecessary, yet you remain timid, avoiding calls and keeping a low profile out of habit. Would you be fair to the relative who paid your debt if you continued to live in fear, as though nothing had been settled?

In the same way, Jesus has fully paid for your healing. The debt has been cleared, and yet many continue to live as if they are still in bondage to sickness, as though the price wasn't paid in full. It wouldn't be fair to Him to carry a burden He already lifted.

This is why divine health is your portion. Embrace it fully, because the sacrifice of Christ not only covered your sins but also secured your healing. Walk in it with confidence, knowing you no longer owe anything to sickness.

You have been healed—by His wounds. Get angry at sickness.

About the Book

"The Seven Keys to Divine Health: Unlocking Your Path to Wholeness" by Emmanuel AnuOluwatomiwa is a practical and inspiring guide to achieving divine health and well-being. This book offers seven essential keys, grounded in biblical principles, to help you maintain physical, emotional, spiritual, and mental health.

Emmanuel provides a clear roadmap for embracing your divine heritage, cultivating a positive mindset, using the power of faith and prayer, and living according to God's laws. Each chapter is filled with personal insights, scriptural teachings, and practical advice for living a life free from sickness and filled with vitality.

Included are powerful scriptural confessions for various health conditions, encouraging you to speak God's healing words over your life daily. Whether you seek healing, wish to maintain a healthy lifestyle, or desire a deeper relationship with God, this book is your guide to living in the fullness of His promises.

Embark on your journey to divine health today with **"The Seven Keys to Divine Health"** and discover how to live a vibrant, faith-filled life.